To Medicate or Not? That Is the Question is definitely honest and insightful in a world full of misinformation and quick fixes. Dr. Asha Pai Bohannon spoke to my sense of duty to my patients and medicine in general. Her pneumonic for H.A.R.M.O.N.Y is both clever and relevant. I honestly hope more people will take their health into their own hands with her advice and research.

– Dr. Mike Harris, M.D.
Board Certified in Family Medicine
Carolina Family Practice & Sports Medicine

Dr. Asha Pai Bohannon has written a clear, concise and up-to-date view on improving blood test results. I truly appreciate her vulnerability and openness in speaking to her own lived experience and journey around healthy lifestyle. Each chapter demonstrates, dissects and illustrates a variety of different techniques to not only improve your blood results, but to improve your overall health. She has done excellent work in speaking to her readers through a holistic lens, with an understanding that not all of her readers are pharmacists or doctors. It is so important to me that people are viewed as a whole, rather than a set of symptoms. The book demonstrates a clear understanding and a need to seek alternative ways of healthy living, when it becomes difficult to find the right answers.

– Dr. Manjunath Burdekar, Psy.D.

Assistant Professor in Psychology at Concord University

To Medicate or Not? That Is the Question is a wonderful source of motivation and support for those looking to take control of their health. Written by a healthcare professional, this book gives the reader a very personal look at what taking the journey out of the health and wellness wilderness can be."

– Dr. Ashley Owens, D.C.

Owner at Carolina Chiropractic

To Medicate or Not? That is the Question!

— TO —
MEDICATE
— OR —
NOT?

That Is *the* Question!

*How to Improve Your Blood Test Results with
the Least Amount of Medication Possible*

Dr. Asha Pai Bohannon
PharmD, CDE, CPT

NEW YORK

LONDON • NASHVILLE • MELBOURNE • VANCOUVER

To Medicate or Not? That is the Question!

How to Improve Your Blood Test Results with the Least Amount of Medication Possible

Published in New York, New York, by Morgan James Publishing in partnership with Difference Press. Morgan James is a trademark of Morgan James, LLC. www.MorganJamesPublishing.com

ISBN 9781642798241 paperback
ISBN 9781642798258 eBook
ISBN 9781642798265 audio
Library of Congress Control Number: 2019950338

Cover Design by:
Rachel Lopez
www.r2cdesign.com

Interior Design by:
Chris Treccani
www.3dogcreative.net

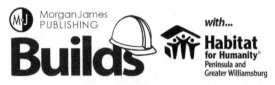

Morgan James is a proud partner of Habitat for Humanity Peninsula and Greater Williamsburg. Partners in building since 2006.

Get involved today! Visit
MorganJamesPublishing.com/giving-back

This book is dedicated to my Mom and Dad. Thank you for being my first two patients and setting the standard for treatment of all my patients. You are my twin pillars of strength; I am so blessed to have been born to you. Thank you for all the sacrifices you have made in life to be able to always support and encourage me. Thank you for showing me that I can do anything I put my mind to and shoot for the stars!

TABLE OF CONTENTS

FOREWORD

In Dr. Asha Pai Bohannon's inaugural work *To Medicate or Not? That is the Question*, she recounts her own struggles with illness and the devastating lack of answers from conventional medicine. She walks the reader along an all too familiar journey through dismissive care, Big Pharma, and the path that ultimately gave her the strength to forge her own way. Through self-exploration, she became the healer she needed, and this empowering book sets out to do the same for the reader. Deftly navigating the gauntlet of emotion so many must face through illness, from self-doubt and frustration to exhaustion and hopelessness, she emerges victorious and beckons for the reader to do the same.

An inventive seven-step program makes an approachable and wholly achievable way to create a foundation of health on which to build for a lifetime. In this way, Dr. Bohannon casts aside the usual stock advice in favor of a comprehensive approach to health and healing fully complementary to conventional medicine when needed.

Arguably, a strong foundation is critical to the efficacy of medical intervention and as such may be implemented by all people, in whatever state of health they may currently be. Adopted by the best and brightest in our field, this kind of whole life approach is the only true personalized medicine and the future of healthcare. Dr. Bohannon's approach empowers all people to achieve what she has done, to take charge of their own well-beings and begin the work of manifesting their own wellness. Ultimately, *To Medicate or Not?* provides a potent life prescription everyone might use; that perhaps our bodies are not battle grounds to fight against but treasures to be honored, heard, and uniquely cared for. I highly recommend it.

Dr. Elizabeth Sierakowski, MD, DABFM
Fellow of Integrative and Functional Medicines
Owner, Essential Health and Wellness Raleigh,
Raleigh, North Carolina
May 2019

INTRODUCTION

Your health shouldn't be all about doctor's visits, prescriptions, and diet programs. It's not a checklist. Your health is a journey; a path that's uniquely yours.

We're not often taught to think this way, but I believe we should be. Your health journey isn't one-size-fits-all, even though the doctors, gurus, and coaches may often dismiss it that way.

For you to move toward a healthier life, what you need to do may be different than someone who's on the same medication or vitamin that you are. A pill, a supplement, an exercise – these things are all powerful, but they aren't the only part of your road ahead that matters. And, in some cases, they don't need to be your first line of treatment.

Too often, focusing on your health is about the medications you need to take, not the life you want to live. But to thrive (not just survive), you need support beyond your medicine cabinet. Because when you want to fix your blood test result numbers, feel more like yourself, find balance, lose weight, or even just have the energy to keep up, you want things that will make a big difference for you. You need personalized solutions that will bring you not just health, but also more hope and harmony into your life.

The reality is that there's so much more to bringing health into your life than what we're told. And you deserve a health journey that will lead you where you want to go, and a guide who can help you at every step of the way. That's exactly why I began my career in healthcare in 2002.

Here's to your Health, Hope, and Harmony in the years to come!

Dr. Asha Pai Bohannon

CHAPTER 1:

The Big
Prescription Push

"The first wealth is health."
– Ralph Waldo Emerson

Have you had your annual physical and been told that several of your blood test results are "off"? Are you too scared to re-test your blood work because you have been told you need to make changes or get on prescriptions the next time the results come in out of range?

If you are anything like me when I got the same results years ago, you are thinking *heck no* I don't want to get on any prescriptions! You may have also tried a million different things that you have seen on social media or found on "Dr.

Google" and nothing has worked. Are you feeling stuck and have no idea what to do?

Let me tell you, I got really tired of hearing "eat less and move more." It left me feeling absolutely hopeless at times and that I would never be able to get healthy, which usually sent me into more of a downward spiral of unhealthy habits. When you feel like you have been working so hard to fix the numbers on your results and nothing is budging, it tends to drain your energy both mentally and physically. You feel like you don't have time for your kids and family or to even think about the things that you enjoy doing. Have you gotten to the point where you have so many things on your plate, that you think, "Well, the things I am doing aren't working, so why spend time on self-care because it just zaps my energy more and I am not getting anywhere?"

When you go back to your healthcare provider, are you telling them you have no idea what to do and their answer is to prescribe medications to bring down the blood work numbers and that will make you feel better? Sometimes this feels like the chicken or the egg scenario. Which comes first – are your results bad because of the way your body is or is your body bad because of how your numbers are? My belief is that if the things that you are seeing work for so many others in your network aren't working for you – it's a deeper issue that won't get fixed with the band-aid solution of prescription medications or quick-fix solutions.

Many other healthcare providers can probably attest to this, but as a pharmacist, we are taught to "First Think Drugs." I believe that the saying means to first think drugs when it comes to possible side effects or interactions. Of course, when I was working in retail pharmacy for many years, the bottom line is usually based off prescription sales. My personal philosophy has always been that the healthier the patient is and feels, the longer they will be a patient.

I'll be honest, I must be seriously keeling over to take a prescription or even an ibuprofen. I do, however, feel like there is a middle ground. There can be a necessity for some prescription use, but it also does not have to be the go-to. There are several other avenues to go down before you rush to prescriptions.

According to a bulletin released by the World Health Organization (WHO) in 2009, there are only two countries in the world that allow direct-to-consumer advertising for pharmaceuticals that include product claims – New Zealand and the United States. This form of advertising has been legal in the USA since 1985, but it started to take off in 1997 when the Food and Drug Administration (FDA) mandated companies to offer the researched indications and a detailed list of side-effects in their ads. Since 1997, the U.S. pharmaceutical industry has focused on and poured money into this form of marketing and advertising. In fact, in 2017 alone, just over six billion dollars was spent on this in the U.S.

An industry group, Pharmaceutical Research and Manufacturers of America (PhRMA), states that the advertising is there to inform patients about their health and treatment options. Dr. Dee Mangin from New Zealand opposes this philosophy and states, "The truth is that direct-to-consumer advertising is used to drive choice rather than inform it," speaking more toward expensive brand-name drugs.

While I agree with Dr. Mangin's statement, "In an era of shared decision-making, it's much more likely that general practitioners will just do what the patient asks;" I have also seen that doctors and other health care professionals aren't just doing what patients ask, they are also being marketed to by the pharmaceutical industry to prescribe their drugs for various reasons, like highlighting the major benefits seen with the new drugs. In fact, marketing dollars for advertising directly toward physicians has increased from over fifteen to over twenty billion dollars between 1997 and 2019. Hence, *The Big Prescription Push!*

What I find is that we are all easily influenced by things we see or hear. We hear a symptom on the TV that sounds like something we have, and we jump to ask about it at our next doctor's visit. How many of you feel ripped off if you go to the doctor's office and don't walk out with a prescription in hand? It seems to be a big trend, because we think we know what is right for ourselves because we see and hear different things all around us. The truth is that we do know our own bodies better than anyone but with all the information that gets literally thrown at us each day, it is very difficult to figure out what is going to work for us.

Wouldn't it be great if you could fix your blood test results with as few prescriptions as possible? If you knew what was right for you and you could then start your journey to a healthier and fuller life? To not feel like something is wrong with you every time you try something to get healthier and it didn't quite work like your friend said it did for them? Wouldn't it be great to not feel hopeless and spiral even further down every time you try something new and it doesn't work?

I completely understand all of those feelings because I was there. I have been working through similar issues for the past ten plus years. You may or may not have heard of this phrase before, but here it is: patient advocacy. Here is a technical definition – a patient advocate helps patients communicate with their healthcare providers, so they get the information they need to make decisions about their healthcare. My role as a patient advocate is all about education and giving you the right information for you, your body, and your healthcare. There is nothing about your health that is one-size-fits-all!

CHAPTER 2:

Not One-Size-Fits-All

*"You are not your illness. You have an individual story
to tell. You have a name, a history, a personality.
Staying yourself is part of the battle."*

– Julian Seifter

Who hasn't been under the impression that what you see
all around you can work for you, too?

I have been in your exact shoes! I absolutely adore my
two boys, but I always tell people that after my second son,
my body decided it was broken and would stay that way until
I figured things out. He is now almost five, and I have spent
the last five years struggling with my own health journey. I am
a holistic health guide and have been for many years. I have
helped people fight their way out of their health struggles and

transform their lives to be able to live the healthy life of their dreams. So, when it came to my own health and wellness, I decided to lean on other healthcare providers and trainers to see me through this process.

Now, when my second son was six months old, I had gotten to a point where I was so fatigued that my immune system was completely shot, and I was sick with some infection or another for ten straight weeks. On top of that, I had gotten to the point that I was so close to falling asleep at the wheel no matter how much sleep I was getting at night. It could have been twelve hours and I would wake up completely exhausted. Want the icing on the cake? My blood work results were all *off!* I started doing what I call "doctor hopping." I was being told I needed to exercise more and eat less; I was being told I needed to get on prescription medications to bring down the numbers; I was being told that I wasn't doing enough and the reason why things I was doing weren't working was because my numbers were off. Now, my numbers never led to an outright diagnosis of anything – they were borderline. But I was working with personal trainer after personal trainer and working with dietitians and healthcare practitioners galore. They would give me regimens to follow and I would follow them to the letter. Guess what happened? *Nada!*

Then from there I started trying various network marketing company products that my friends were selling that seemed to have great results for others based on before and after pictures. Nothing ever worked. Now, I am not saying they don't work or are not good because I saw amazing results for others and did research the products before using them. I just didn't get results myself. So, I moved on to popular nutrition plans I was hearing about: Whole 30, Keto diet, Paleo…. You name it, I probably tried it. Several of those my supportive husband even did with me. He (as thin as he already is) would even lose fifteen or so pounds in a thirty-day period, and me (who on top of fixing my blood tests had a bit of weight to lose) struggled to get five pounds off in the same month.

I knew at this point there was more to it. I went back to the drawing board – my general physician. He sent me to a specialist – an endocrinologist. This endocrinologist looked at my past lab results (which were all slightly elevated or away from normal) and told me I was pre-diabetic and that was my problem. She said I needed to eat less and work out more (definitely heard that more than my fair share of times in the past). She then prescribed me a drug used for most Type 2 Diabetes patients called Metformin. Being a pharmacist, I know what the normal dose of this medication for a newly diagnosed diabetes patient should be. Remember,

I was not diabetic – just had slightly elevated blood sugars. She prescribed a dose three times that of a starting dose for a newly diagnosed diabetic, then had me pay out of pocket for some elaborate scanning tests (for which they didn't even put in the right patient information). I felt completely scammed by all of this. But, moving onward and focusing on my health issues.... Since I happen to know the dose of the prescription was *way too high*, and the major side effect of lactic acidosis (a buildup of lactic acid in the body which occurs when cells make lactic acid from glucose faster than it can be metabolized) that can occur with this medication, I went ahead and cut the dose in half. Within thirty minutes of me taking the half dose, I couldn't move my entire body and it stayed that way for the next four hours. I was in massive pain. I tried it again the next day to make sure it wasn't a fluke; of course, it happened again. I don't even want to imagine what might have happened if I ended up taking the dose the doctor originally prescribed. From there I went back to my primary care physician's office and spoke to a physician's assistant. She then gave me a prescription for an injection that helps lower insulin resistance which is a sign for pre-diabetes, plus it has a positive side effect of losing some weight. Feeling hopeless and desperate, I was pulling at strings to bring down my blood test results, get this weight off *and* feel better, I decided to go ahead and try it. Low and behold, I had major allergic reactions with red, itchy spots all over the injection sites. After six weeks of struggling like that, guess what? *Nada!* Quite honestly, at that point, I got tired of being told I was a *"medical mystery"* and being dismissed from every practice I tried.

So several years, providers, thousands of dollars later, and all the hard work I had done, my blood test results began to look "normal." Yay! Right? Nope. After all that, I was still feeling like death warmed over daily, still exhausted, still fighting weight loss resistance. I started looking at blood work testing and what is "normal." Here is what I found – when you look at the "normal" ranges on any given lab work from a typical physical, the ranges are very large – most people will fall within these ranges of normal. So, what happens if you are still having symptoms and don't have results outside of range?

I found a physician that was willing to listen to my symptoms and dig a little deeper. We started looking at my thyroid because I was having several symptoms of hypothyroidism, but my thyroid numbers were within the "normal" range. My physician and I decided it was worth a try to start me on a low-dose thyroid medication to see if I might have a subclinical (symptoms with lab results being in normal range) form of thyroid disorder and if that would spark my metabolism to kick in. I was on that for about four months and at that time I had gotten into a very regimented, rigorous exercise routine. I was starting to see small weight loss. Yay! After the four months, I talked to my physician to see if we could stop the medication and see if I could continue the weight loss on my own with the lifestyle regimen I was doing. He agreed, and during the year, as my personal life became way too stressful to talk about here, and the stopping of the thyroid med, the weight loss plateaued and eventually the weight came back on slowly despite the same rigorous regimen I was doing. Then I got back on the thyroid med to see if that really was the issue and instead of losing weight this time – weight came pouring on with a vengeance.

My physician was completely stumped. As I said before, throughout the years I heard "you are a medical mystery" and this physician was no different – he said the exact same thing. I then got sent to another specialist, who long story short, told me he would see me through this process and make sure to help me figure out what was wrong. After one set of tests that came back negative – he had his nurse call me and "dismiss" me from his practice. I was completely appalled!

A valuable concept that became clearer and clearer through all of this is that every *body* is different and will react differently to different medications, regimens, and lifestyle changes. I was never a fan of being on any prescription medications unless absolutely necessary. I have always been completely against the band-aid approach to health issues, but now that I had already given in, and tried a couple out of desperation, and then experienced the awful side effects for myself – I knew for sure just how opposed I was. I knew deep down there had to be another issue going on. Why wasn't I able to lose weight despite all the efforts? Why wasn't I able to get my energy back despite all the efforts?

Where did that leave me? I have always told my husband that I absolutely *love* helping others find the right information that works for their bodies and making sure they are knowledgeable with what's relevant to them. The ironic thing was I was truly searching for someone out there to do the same thing for me that I do for others, I was looking for a "*me* for *me*"! The concept of patient advocacy kept popping up in my head over and over. In this day and age of media at our fingertips, gathering information can be done at the blink of an eye. Turn on the TV and you hear several symptoms that you may be experiencing. Click an app on your phone and the image of someone getting results that you want may pop up. Or if nothing else, type what you are searching for into a search engine. The problem comes from not knowing whether or not "Dr. Google" is giving you the right information for *You!* Knowing what is right for you and then being able to speak to your healthcare provider with the right information can help to improve your health outcomes, reduce your healthcare spending, and help improve your quality of life.

As I started to realize that there was an overwhelming amount of information out there, and that many providers just do not have the time to spend sifting through all of it for each individual, something needed to be done. Someone needed to be that missing link between the information available, the providers, and the patients. So, I delved into all of this and created the method that is going to be laid out over the next few chapters and have found the answers to my own life and health concerns along the way!

CHAPTER 3:

Less Medications, More Results – 7 Steps to H.A.R.M.O.N.Y.™

"Health is a state of complete harmony
of the body, mind, and spirit."
– B.K.S. Iyengar

As discussed in the last chapter, our health is not one-size-fits-all. With all the information we have at our fingertips these days, it feels like what we see everyone else doing should work for us too. There is more direct-to-consumer advertising and more comparison then there ever used to be pre-internet and social media. Not only are we thinking that these things we see should be working for us too, but if they don't work, we beat ourselves up over the fact that it doesn't work and we aren't seeing results. Do you start to blame yourself for it not working? Do you start to ask what is wrong with you? Do you get into a downward spiral of negative thoughts about yourself? What we should be asking is "*Why* is this not working and what am I truly missing about myself and my body?"

My entire practice is based on the patient advocacy concept. It starts with digging to find out more and more information about you as an individual and your past. Then we dig deeper to find out what is going on in your body and your mind in the present moment to then be able to provide the right recommendations to help you soar into your healthy future!

For years I have struggled with the concept of finding *balance* in my life – as a wife, mom, daughter, professional/entrepreneur, PTA parent, caregiver – and about what feels like fifty other hats. What is balance? Balance is something that is often mentioned in personal development and well-being circles. It is said you should eat a balanced diet, live a balanced life, and seek a good work/family balance. When I hear this, I start to visualize Chinese acrobats spinning several plates on tiny poles and keeping them balanced so they don't fall. That is a very precise and unbelievably difficult task that very few people in this world can do. One misstep and all the plates can come crashing down. Well, the way I see it – life is full of missteps. So, what happens when the plates come crashing down? If you are like most people, you start to come down hard on yourself and you spend most of your life wondering how to have it all and make it all work at the same time, as life whizzes by you in a blur. We add more and more "plates to our poles" and if it doesn't work the way we think, or we end up doing half the job we think we should do – that negative voice starts to come blaring out at you.

To be honest, I don't like the word *balance*. It has such a negative connotation these days. We beat ourselves up and question on a daily basis why we can't find balance in our lives. So, I use the word *harmony*. This concept of living your life in harmony means that you *can* have it all, and you *can* be it all, just not at the same time and in the way our surroundings are telling us we should be. Harmony is about finding the people, activities, and emotions that are suitable for ourselves and the type of life we want to lead. It's about knowing that we don't have to balance a thousand plates without letting them fall. It's about doing one thing at a time, doing it well and living in the moment of what we are doing.

The only way to truly live in harmony is to get a full 360-degree view of your life and see how everything we do affects our health. We have to stop letting our surroundings dictate what we "should" be doing. In this chapter, I will give you an overview of the process I use to do just that. My 7 Steps to H.A.R.M.O.N.Y. includes:

- H – Healthy History – Comprehensive Assessment
- A – Analysis of Medication/ Supplement profile and Lab results
- R – Realizing that your Journey is Unique
- M – Maximizing your Physical Attributes
- O – Opportunities for Internal Growth
- N – Nurture Your Stress Relief
- Y – You have the P.O.W.E.R. to Transform Your Life

All you need is the right information to guide you in the right direction for you as an individual. By working through this process, you will get your blood work results back down to normal and as a nice benefit – find your sense of purpose and feel more energized while feeling the healthiest you have ever felt. Are you ready to lead your healthiest life yet and be the person you have always dreamt of being? How about getting to that point on the least amount of medications/ supplements necessary and the right lifestyle change guidance to suit your needs and desires? Well, let's get started!

CHAPTER 4:

Step 1 – Health History –
Comprehensive Assessment

"Study the past if you would define the future."
– Confucius

W hy do we start with your history? A complete and accurate history is the foundation to helping decide how to proceed with the future of your health journey. We must know where you have come from and know what has been done, in order to know where to go.

Often times when our health is at risk and/ or we feel awful, we tend to do what I call provider hop to search for answers and get the answers we think we want. Another thing we tend to do is ask "Dr. Google" for the answers of what to do. So to begin, we need to get a thorough account of what has happened in your history, and what you have done when it comes to labs, medications, supplements, nutrition, and exercise. We spend quite a bit of time digging into all of this as well as the philosophies that you have and what you are willing and not willing to do for your health. We discuss your current symptoms, and what *all* of your ultimate goals for your health are (including getting those blood work numbers down). We dig deep into what you have been told by your providers and what has worked and what hasn't.

We address the fear of not wanting to take medications and how sometimes they can be necessary, but we will do everything we can to steer clear of them. We talk thoroughly about the symptoms that you have experienced and what is currently going on. A lot of times we go to providers and hear the same "eat less, exercise more" mantra or they say to "take this prescription to bring down the numbers and you will feel better." Essentially it is a band-aid solution to stop the issue for a while – only to see that you aren't getting anywhere in your health goals. While you might feel better for a short period of time, you end up feeling just as bad or even worse after the band-aid falls off.

Clearly there is a deeper issue going on and you need someone that is willing to take the time to listen to what you need and dig deeper with you to find the right answers for you. Western medicine and our society today have a thought process that there is a "magic pill" or quick fix for everything; I don't blame anyone for that because I have certainly been in that position. We are a society of wanting results now, convenience, and going after what we want in the easiest ways possible. The problem with all of this is that there is no magic pill and if we go for the quick fix it almost always backfires on us. It can provide some relief but if you have not gotten to the root of the problem, then you have not fixed the cause and it will almost always come back and may even manifest in a different way. This different way usually spurs a provider to add yet another medication to your growing list to deal with a "separate issue," when in fact if you had dealt with the original problem to begin with, it may have never come up again. That is why we start with a detailed history of what other programs you have tried in the past and you tell me what has worked and what has not. This is so we know what not to try again and waste anyone's time, energy, or money.

Another reason for a thorough health history is because when you start to talk through what you have gone through and what you are feeling at that moment, more things will come up that have never come up before. Often times we are so focused on the external or what we see. The blood work numbers are in front of us and so that is where our attention goes. Once we start opening up about what has been happening, we discover many other facets of our lives that contribute to health issues that go way beyond the numbers.

Looking at past labs can give us an indication of what has been done so we can figure out the next steps and what else needs to be looked at.

Going a little further back, even with all the technology we have at our disposal today, it is still our own family history and past experiences that shape how our health looks today and can look in the future.

Family History: How does it help?

- It's a tool to help identify risks and can aid in diagnosis.
- It's a tool to help make informed decisions about screening, patient education, and other preventative health measures.
- It's a tool to help providers understand family relationships and identify environments and behaviors that might put a patient at higher risk for certain diseases.
- It's a tool to help identify genetic patterns.

- It's a tool to help correct misguided beliefs – for example, that a disease affects only one gender or skips a generation.

A thorough family history is also vitally important because sometimes things are out of our control. This means that no matter how hard we work or how hard we dig; the numbers just won't change because the family history is so strong.

Your genetic makeup is not something you can change. Risks for diseases like asthma, diabetes, cancer, and heart disease run in families. But knowing your family history can decrease the risk of developing health problems or prolong their impact on your own life. The other piece to it is that family members not only share their genes, but also their lifestyles, habits, and environment.

What trends are we looking for in Family History?

- Disease in more than one close relative
- Diseases that don't usually affect a certain gender (i.e., breast cancer in males)
- Diseases occurring at an earlier age than expected (i.e., 10-20 years before)

• Combinations of diseases in relatives (i.e., both breast and ovarian cancer or heart disease and diabetes)

My mom has a very strong family history of Type 2 Diabetes (her mother, sister, and younger brother). She was always aware of this, especially since her own mother passed away at the very young age of fifty-two from complications of uncontrolled diabetes. Knowing that the likelihood of developing diabetes herself was extremely high, she did an incredible job of taking care of herself and running her life the way that works for her over the years. She was not diagnosed with overt diabetes until she was fifty years old. She would not have been able to prolong that diagnosis if she went through life not knowing what her history was like.

During this process, we get to know each other much better and truly begin to feel comfortable with one another. We dig deep into your goals for your health beyond just bringing the numbers down. This process is for more than just that – it's about you getting to live a healthy life of your dreams and maintaining it. We need to know what that truly looks like for you.

CHAPTER 5:

Step 2 – Analyze Medication/ Supplement Profile and Lab Testing

"Polypharmacy increases the risk of adverse reactions to medications. The more drugs, the higher the risk of drug interactions."

– U.S. Pharmacist, June 16, 2017

What is polypharmacy? Polypharmacy is defined as the concurrent use of multiple medications by a single patient to treat one or more conditions. There are several reasons why this happens:

- *Prescribing Cascades:* If you have several health conditions, you may be given a prescription to counteract side effects of another medication or to counteract an interaction between two or more other prescribed medications.

- *Disconnected medical care:* This is more likely to occur if you are cared for by several doctors, including specialists or short-term hospitalizations. One doctor may give you a prescription that counteracts the effect of a medication you already take, particularly if you are getting care at a different healthcare center than usual. Also, if you are in a short-term care facility, providers can start you on a medication intended for short-term use and once you leave it may be refilled continuously by your primary physician because they did not know that the original indication was for short-term use.

- *Pharmacy changes:* If you fill your prescriptions at multiple pharmacies, none are likely to have a complete list of your medication regimen. Interactions between medications may go unnoticed unlike if you get all of your medications from the same place.

- *Direct-to-Consumer Advertising:* A large part of polypharmacy issues comes from this advertising practice.

- *Band-aid Effect:* In emergent situations, providers don't always have all the information, so the typical practice is to put band-aids on the situation. For example, recently we had to take my dad to the emergency room for an extremely swollen foot with a lot of pain and redness. We were worried it was a clot. After running two different tests, the physician determined that it wasn't a clot. But he then made the comment that the tests were "inconclusive." So, after a five-hour stay in the E.R., he decided he would send my dad home with a prescription for an acute gout attack and an antibiotic for possible cellulitis infection (a bacterial skin infection). After we received the prescriptions, I was shocked that he chose an antibiotic that is usually only prescribed if a patient has allergies to the first line of treatment and a dose that was triple the normal dose. In addition, one of the main side effects for this medication is a more severe gut infection. How this physician could have prescribed that for an eighty-three-year old man with a *possible* infection that had no evidence that is what it was, it horrified me. We did not get it filled we went back to my dad's primary care physician and figured out the diagnosis and care plan. It absolutely terrifies me that this practice is the "norm" in our healthcare system.

A large part of these polypharmacy issues come from our countries allowance of direct-to-consumer advertising (discussed in an earlier chapter). What I am getting at is, we see/ hear something on TV or Social Media and think "I have what they are describing," we go into the doctor's office and describe our symptoms and say I saw a commercial for this prescription and a lot of the times the provider says, "Ok, let's give it a try." With very little follow-up, it is difficult to see if the prescription is even working or perhaps it causes another problem from a side effect. When you go back in after a while with a new symptom (perhaps to a different provider), the provider doesn't always take a look or know what you are on or what the interactions or adverse effects might be. So they begin to treat the symptom you are currently complaining about. And this process continues until you end up way worse off than you started to begin with.

In this step, we get a very detailed account of every prescription, nutritional or herbal supplement, and/or over-the-counter medication that you have taken during this entire process. We will go over what they were for, how they made you feel, and if any of them worked and provided the results that were explained to you. The idea behind this profile is to get you on as few prescription medications as possible and see if the band-aid effect discussed in the last chapter and above has been occurring so much that it ends up being a detriment and causing more issues for you.

Another example of the band-aid effect, I had a patient who had several conditions and ended up on a total of fifteen prescription medications, and several nutritional supplements to combat issues. After digging deeper into this, we found out that as time had passed, more and more prescriptions were being prescribed because new symptoms would pop up or things seemed to be getting worse. He ended up contacting me because instead of feeling better this forty-five-year old (once vibrant) male was beginning to feel frail and out of sorts often and his activities of daily living were diminishing. He "just couldn't function like he used to." He described the symptoms he was currently experiencing and explained a very thorough health history – his current medication profile was then analyzed for interactions, side effects, and duplications. We found that more and more prescriptions were being piled on as a result of him going to his provider for new symptoms. To complicate the issues, these prescriptions that got added on while trying to "fix" new issues that arose (from side effects) were actually interacting with the original medications (that were causing the side effects in the first place) for the diseases – this in turn was causing a whole other syndrome with a whole host of other symptoms. After doing extensive research and finding alternatives to the original medications that were causing problems but were necessary, I was able to provide research-backed recommendations that the patient agreed with and could then take to his primary care provider and "fight" to get back his health. The physician agreed to the recommendations and within three weeks I received an email telling me that he hadn't felt this good in ten years.

What this story shows is that we are a band-aid society. We think that symptoms come from the original issue, or the fact that the blood work is off, but when we dig a little deeper the origin could be somewhere we never expected or thought of to begin with.

Another example of this is when a sixty-year-old female had been diagnosed with a not-so-common liver issue. She had done some "Dr. Google" searching and was able to find a little bit of information as to why certain liver test results were off. Upon doing the research, I was able to find another medication that helps to specifically lower the specific lab result that was elevated. As I mentioned before, in some cases there is no way around prescriptions, and they can be necessary. This new prescription had a side effect of itching. After looking at what she had been prescribed prior to this – she was placed on another less effective prescription for the same reason that also had severe itching as a potential side effect. She had tolerated that one fine but was worried about adding another medication to it with the same side effect. When looking at the dosing, I noticed she had been prescribed (and taking) double the maximum dose of this medication. She mentioned that her provider had kept increasing the dose to see if that would bring down the blood results, and even though it hadn't, she had been taking this massive dose for over a year with no help to her results. She mentioned she kept taking it without question because it was what her physician told her. Now, I am not here to tell you not to listen to your providers. It's about knowing what and why you are taking prescriptions and the effect they can have on you. After I gave specific recommendations and they were accepted by her physician, the patient was able to decrease the original prescription, add the new one, and ultimately bring down the blood results that were of concern to begin with – and with no side effects.

Another consideration with medications is our age. As we age and diseases progress or just the natural band-aid effect occurs, the chances of taking more and more medications increases. Aging changes our bodies which can modify how we are able to process medications, how they are absorbed, and how they are utilized. We also become more sensitive to medications. So, prescriptions can stay in our bodies longer and decrease vital organ function (i.e., the liver and kidneys) which can increase side effects, drug interactions, and other adverse drug reactions.

On top of prescription medication issues, our current lifestyles and habits and our genes can cause us to have certain deficiencies. Our bodies are meant to have a certain amount of vitamins/ minerals/ nutrients. Technically, if we ate the way we are meant to eat, we should be able to get all that we need through the nutritious foods around us. However, let's go back to the society of convenience as I mentioned before. What we are finding is that there are a lot of people getting health issues causing deficiencies in their bodies because they are just not eating like they should be, or the foods they eat are not what they once were. I must stop here because that may be a whole other book topic. The good news is that now we have access to look at several types of lab test panels that can show deficiencies that may be going on in your body based on what we are currently doing and in what conditions our genes would react best, in order to help address the root issues that are causing your symptoms. More about these tests will be discussed in the next chapter.

Once getting the information about any deficiencies, how do you know what supplements are right for you when you can walk into any corner drugstore and find dozens of different brands? When you go to a provider that specializes in medication management and holistic healthcare, you know they are looking at the manufacturing processes, what types of ingredients and fillers are being used and you can feel confident that you are getting what you are told you are getting.

As you can see, it becomes a vicious cycle. There are alternatives to how you can treat certain issues that arise. Knowing what to discuss and bring up with your provider is a *key component* on your health journey.

CHAPTER 6:

Step 3 – Realizing Your Journey Is Unique

"While the same physical mechanisms and the same metabolic processes are operating in all human bodies, the structures are sufficiently diverse [that] the sum total of all the reactions taking place in one individual's body may be very different from those taking place in the body of another individual of same age, sex, and body size."

– Dr. Roger J. Williams

A re you being told your blood work is off because you need to lose the excess weight? Here is the reason why you hear this. The National Institutes of Health states that a twenty-pound weight loss can lower blood pressure by five to twenty points in the systolic number (top number). And John Hopkins Medicine states that lowering your body weight by five to ten percent can lower your risk of developing diabetes by fifty-eight percent. While this is great information and things to aim for, it works for some and not for everyone. Just focusing on the weight loss by any means necessary can work for some, and results can be transformational – but are they lasting? I have all too many times seen people do the latest and greatest fad that is out there and get results. But once they stop doing what they were doing they go back to where they were. Others can try and try using some of the same programs and come out on the other end in the same place or worse off than when they started. What does all this mean? It means that we are all *unique!* It means that our health and wellness is not cookie-cutter. For the first person that gets results from these programs but goes right back to square one, we need to find something that is sustainable for that person that matches what his/her goals are and what that person is or is not willing to do for their health long-term. For the second person that is not able to get results from these programs, first, they can often feel like a failure and get dejected by not getting any results. They can't seem to figure out why and often times they spiral out of control making their results and symptoms worse than before. For these patients, we have to dig deeper into their biochemistry and look at a 360-degree view of that person and fix what is missing or gone awry in their lives.

As seen a lot today on social media, we are given the misconception that if we follow a certain plan or regimen that our results will be the same as the many before and after pictures we see and the stories we read about. We are under the impression that following that meal plan, or that specific exercise routine, or taking that certain supplement or prescription can solve our blood work issues, drop that weight, or give back that energy we are so longing to fix. Or, we are given the misconception that we can do things without prescriptions and completely "naturally" or with certain supplements. All may be true, and I am not discounting that you do not always have to take prescriptions to get the results you want, but if you follow what someone else's results have gotten them, it does not always equate to giving you the results you need or want or it could be the wrong type for you and your body.

Now, let's talk about prescription medications. Yes, they are made for the general public, but as we all know, side effects are always reported in any clinical trial done for these medications. Why is that? Because biochemically we are all individuals.

I shared my own experience with this in Chapter 2. Here is another example of my own dad's prescription mishap. About five years ago, I was about ready to pop with my second child. My dad limped into my house to help with something and I could tell he could barely walk. Now, he was only on two prescription medications (one for a family cholesterol issue and one for high blood pressure) and had been for twenty plus years with no problems to speak of. He had been a very active and healthy man up to that point. When I inquired about what was going on, he brushed it off as nothing, just a little pain in his feet. Then after inquiring a bit further, he mentioned it had been a growing problem for about a year and half. His feet had been swelling and progressively getting worse over time. He said he told his physician about it and was given another two new prescriptions to combat the swelling. The doctor explained that it was because he was aging and more problems/diseases were starting to come up. From the addition of those two medications, the original problem of the swelling feet clearly was not being helped and he was starting to have other issues arise due to the new meds.

I dug a little deeper and discovered that while his two prescriptions were doing just fine and he was not having any concerns – his provider switched him to a newer blood pressure medication about a year and a half ago just before his feet started to swell. After researching the prescription that he was switched to, there was a report of a one percent chance that people could get edema in the lower extremities (swelling in the feet). At that point, I contacted the provider and let him know about this chance and what was going on with my dad. He brushed it off and said, "That's only a one percent chance." I then asked the provider, "What if my dad is in that one percent?" Without changing anything else, I recommended we go back to his original medication for blood pressure for one week. I would monitor his blood pressure numbers and if there is a problem at all, we could switch him back to whatever the doctor recommends. He agreed.

Let me tell you – my dad's feet went back to completely normal within three days and he was able to stop the other two extra prescriptions he was put on as a result of the swelling. What does all this mean? You are an individual and things can happen that are not common, and we have to look at you and your symptoms as a problem to solve, not just to band-aid. It turned out the pharmaceutical rep for that new drug had just come into the office a few weeks before my dad had been in. The doctor was told all the wonderful aspects of this new medication and decided to change my dad to it even though there was no issues with what he was on.

Now, let's talk digging deeper biochemically! Your lab results are unique to you. We like to play the comparison game in everything we do, but when it comes to your own blood work – there is no comparison. That being said, the normal complete blood panel you get when you go to a general provider can tell you some information but is usually a snapshot. It measures your blood plasma/serum and can tell you a 4-72-hour snapshot of what you have done. Sometimes people will "shape up" what they are doing in that timeframe if they know they are having tests done. These are great ways to see a certain period of time to see what may be going on.

Going back to my story, I knew I had already gotten the common blood panels done a million times. So, I went to a more natural-based doctor who dug deeper into the blood work panels. After getting a ton of that blood work done, she ended up giving me several supplements to fix the various results that came up. I was put on one thing for gut issues, several things for blood sugar issues, and several things for adrenal issues *all at the same time*. The problem here was instead of focusing on one particular issue at a time and finding the root cause, I felt like she was band-aiding the issues – this time with supplements and not prescriptions as was done before by other practitioners. Result = none!

What I have discovered over the years that needs to happen is to (1) figure out the underlying cause, and (2) focus attention on that particular issue for a period of time before moving to the next issue. The question I always like to ask first is: What is the underlying cause of the condition? After looking at the health and family history, the next clues are on a cellular and genetic level. Did you know there is a way to have your own individual cellular function measured? This testing can go beyond the normal panels you get at a physical. It allows your provider to guide your journey toward preventing diseases, wellness, aging management, and slowing cellular dysfunction – all by targeting defined nutritional deficiencies and genetic make-up.

Examples of the testing available:

- Micronutrient testing
- Epigenetic testing
- Cardiometabolic panel
- Hormone panel
- Various genetic markers/mapping (i.e., genetic variants, telomere length, MTHFR)

Micronutrient and epigenetic testing are a more precise way to look at you as an individual and find out what makes your body tick. With micronutrient testing we get a snapshot of your current nutrient levels. When we look at the intracellular space vs. the plasma/serum, it helps you see how your cells are handling different vitamins and minerals. For example, folic acid measurements from the serum is not going to be fully telling because folic acid has no business in the serum, its function is actually inside the cell. With epigenetic testing we see how your genes respond, not only to your environment, but also to your lifestyle choices. We can be eating what we think is the healthiest foods but may not be able to absorb the nutrients properly or getting enough for our own bodies' needs. How is it that one person can eat certain foods and not gain weight, while another can eat the exact same foods and struggle with their weight? These tests can let us know any deficiencies that might be causing problems and we can know exactly how we need to adjust your nutrition and/or supplements.

CHAPTER 7:

Step 4 – Maximizing Your Physical

"We only need to focus on the things we have control over. It is a waste of time and energy to worry about the things in our life that we have absolutely no control over. No matter how much you worry, the things that are supposed to happen will happen."

– Kasturi Pai (my mom)

I used to be a big worrier when I was younger, but I still can hear my mom telling me the quote above. For example, when I would complain to her about my professor in college being extremely tough and I probably would not pass an exam, she would tell me, "You can't control the professor or how he/she grades, the only thing you have control over is how much work you do and how hard you study the materials. If you don't do that, then the only person you can blame is yourself if you don't pass." Here are some things that you don't have control over: other people's actions, other people's feelings, other people's opinions, and other people's mistakes. What you do have control over: your attitude, your effort, your behavior, and your actions.

The same thing holds true when it comes to our health and wellness. Every *body* is different. Let's take weight loss for example. Have you ever heard someone say, "I just had to cut out drinking sodas and I dropped twenty pounds," and you are thinking "I already cut out sodas and have lost hardly anything!" We don't have control over how our body responds to certain things we do, but we do have control over *what* we do. We know that cutting out those regular sodas is affecting our bodies in a good way to some degree. But let's take this a little further.... What other things do we have control over that we can work on? Our nutrition, our activity level, the amount of rest we get on a daily basis, and how much we stay hydrated. We are going to touch on each one of these and why it's so important that we do the things that match our own bodies. Yes, we can try the dreaded four-letter word D-I-E-T or cookie-cutter programs that are out there, but are they sustainable, are they right for your body, and will they work? As I mentioned in my story before, I am a prime example. I tried umpteen different well-advertised programs (this shake, these supplements) and drooled over every before and after picture, but to no avail. It was not until I started customizing my nutrition, my exercise plan and focusing on the amount of rest and hydration I was getting daily, that I started getting results I needed in order to decrease my own blood work numbers, even start seeing weight loss results, and gaining back the energy I needed to lead the life I had hoped for.

Nutrition

If we have poor nutrition, or do not get the adequate amounts of the nutrients our bodies need, it allows chronic inflammation to start in our bodies. (Look for more information about inflammation in Chapter 9.)

The first controllable place to start on any health journey is to evaluate your nutrition and make the necessary changes to what you are doing immediately. Cut out processed foods, stick to whole, natural, and nutritious foods. Be sure to include a wide variety of fruits and vegetables. I could sit and name several popular diets and products out there right now, but I don't like calling those types of things out. Instead, I will be honest with my thoughts, I am not a fan of exclusion diets, and so many fad diets these days are just that – they cut out essential macronutrients that our body does need, for long periods of time. I believe where we go wrong is by the types of foods we are consuming and how they are made in our society today.

So how do you figure out what's right for you? There are several ways, as explained earlier, there is micronutrient and epigenetic testing we can do. In addition, another method I use and learned about from my training with the International Association of Wellness Professionals is body typing. Body typing is a way of living that provides guidelines on nutrition, exercise, behavior and overall health based on physical, mental, and emotional characteristics. There are three main Body Types (Doshas), and even though we are all a combination of all three, we tend to show dominance in one over the rest. ©The Get Real Plan, 2011-2012 has created a quiz to discover your body type. In order to take this quiz, please go to ashapaibohannon.com for a copy of the quiz and explanations about each Dosha.

Exercise

According to the Guidelines for Adults created by the Department of Health and Human Services (revised in 2018):

- Adults should move more and sit less throughout the day. Some physical activity is better than none.

Adults who sit less and do any amount of moderate-to-vigorous physical activity gain some health benefits. There are passive, active and integrated ways to get in activity:

- o Passive: walking or playing with the dog; taking a walk, hike, or jog; swimming; riding a bicycle or rollerblading
- o Active: training for a race; joining a running club, swim team, cycling club; joining a recreational sports team
- o Integrated: walking around the office more frequently; household chores (being more rigorous); biking or walking to places; parking further away in a parking lot
- For substantial health benefits, adults should do at least 150 minutes to 300 minutes a week of moderate-intensity, or 75 minutes to 150 minutes a week of vigorous-intensity aerobic physical activity. Aerobic activity should be spread throughout the week.
- Additional health benefits are gained by engaging in physical activity beyond the equivalent of 300 minutes of moderate-intensity physical activity a week.

- Adults should also do muscle-strengthening activities of moderate or greater intensity and that involve all major muscle groups on two or more days a week.

Jogging/running, swimming, cycling? Strength training? Zumba, dancing, boxing? What tickles your fancy when it comes to exercise? I always say the best activity is the one that you will do. However, what I see a lot is people doing the same exercises as everyone else they see. Just like with nutrition – there are certain types of exercise that may work better for you than others. Training for a half marathon may have weight loss effects on one person and may not have any weight loss benefits for another person. I am definitely proof of this one! I love running, and I have trained for two half marathons. I bought the training books, found a four-month running and nutrition regimen to follow – which I followed to the letter (I am a compliant patient). Happily, I was able to complete the two races (running the entire courses); however, none of my efforts led to weight loss. This is an example of how there is either a deeper issue or how your genes can play a role in what types of exercise your body will respond to. We can get this information by using epigenetic testing.

The other piece people tend to forget is our bodies can become tolerant to types of foods we eat and exercises we do if we do them every day or on a regular basis. So, we have to switch things up and be aware of any restrictions that your body is telling you. My advice is to work with a certified personal trainer to determine what's right for you.

Hydration

The proper amount of hydration has amazing benefits for you, such as:

- Increases brain power and provides energy
- Promotes healthy weight management and weight loss
- Flushes out toxins
- Improves your complexion
- Maintains regularity
- Boosts immune system
- Prevents headaches
- Prevents cramps and sprains.

Now that we know what hydrating ourselves can do, let's talk about how much we need to get:

1. Take your current weight (in pounds) and divide that number by two.

2. Optional: Add 32 ounces to that number (to get an added boost of hydration through the day)
3. Your total is how many ounces of water you should drink each day. You can divide that number by eight to see how many cups you need to drink each day.

What drinks constitute proper hydration?

Water! Not a surprise, right? It is the *number one best way to hydrate yourself* (But if you just can't stomach water all day long, here are some good alternatives):

- Milk (Added bonus: it has calcium and vitamin D, and protein to keep you fueled on even the hottest of days; one thing to think about here is the inflammatory effects of dairy if that is of concern for your body)
- Fruit-infused water (If plain water is hard to stomach, infusing your water with fruit is a healthy way to add flavor without adding sugar. Examples: lime and basil, lemon with raspberry, or cucumber with mint)
- Watermelon (I know this isn't a drink and watermelon does have a high sugar content so if you are diabetic you have to be super careful with portion control, but every time you eat watermelon, you're holding onto ninety-two percent of the liquid you're eating.)

- Teas (Caffeine-free and herbal teas are the best options. Tea is also packed with antioxidants. Avoid caffeine in general, it's a diuretic, meaning it dehydrates!)
- Coconut water (Contains ninety-five percent water; check the label for hidden sugar content)
- Milk alternatives like soy, coconut, and almond (from the right sources)
- When it comes to drinks other than water, as is with everything in life – moderation is key!

Ok, just to keep harmony with the good vs. bad, let's just list the beverages that made the naughty list:

- Soda (has dehydrating caffeine, and a lot of sugar and sodium which also retain water)
- Beer/wine/liquor (any kind of alcohol removes water from your tissues which increases the need to drink more water to replace it; it also provides extra calories and carbohydrates which can be stored as triglycerides/ fats)
- Hot cocoa (Contains more sugar and calories than a can of soda – can lead to dehydration)

- Coffee (In moderation, coffee isn't too bad, but once you go past that second cup, your body really starts to suffer. Drinking more than 200-300 milligrams of caffeine (the amount in two to three cups of coffee) has been shown to lead to dehydration. To keep yourself safe, switch to decaf if you're a heavy coffee drinker, or limit yourself to a cup or two; Another consideration- black coffee has benefits, but we have to be careful with adding any creamer or sugar/ sugar substitute.)
- Lemonade (high sugar content)
- Sweet tea (high sugar content and caffeine)
- Energy drinks (Filled with caffeine, sugars and chemicals)
- Flavored milks (Avoid chocolate, strawberry, and vanilla)
- Smoothies (Certain homemade smoothies can be good for you, but you have to be careful with the types of fruits you use and commercial made smoothies, especially the ones you don't know the ingredients for)

Rest

> *"Early to bed and early to rise makes a man*
> *healthy, wealthy, and wise."*
> **– Benjamin Franklin**

If you are anything like I used to be, you run on fumes all the time because you always have "something" to get done. The problem is that if you continue to run on fumes and do not allow your body to rest and rejuvenate, ill-health effects start to happen. Not getting enough rest can have the following impact:

- Weakened immune system
- Increased risk of respiratory diseases
- Increased weight loss resistance (two hormones leptin and ghrelin, control feelings of hunger and satiety; sleep deprivation also increases the release of insulin which leads to increased fat storage)
- Increased blood pressure, sugar levels, inflammation
- Decreased hormone production (including growth hormone, as we age growth hormone helps increase muscle mass and thickens skin and strengthen bones, and testosterone)

- Affected alertness and concentration (cognitive thinking)
- Affected libido
- Affected mood (can lead to signs of depression)
- Aging your skin (puffy eyes, and cortisol which is a hormone released in response to lack of sleep breaks down collagen)
- Affected memory and judgment ability

Now that we know how lack of sleep/rest can affect our health, how much rest is good for your health? According to the National Sleep Foundation (NSF) 2015 recommendations for appropriate sleep durations for specific age groups are:

- Newborns (0 to 3 months): 14 to 17 hours each day
- Infants (4 to 11 months): 12 to 15 hours
- Toddlers (1 to 2 years): 11 to 14 hours
- Preschoolers (3 to 5 years): 10 to 13 hours
- School-age children (6 to 13 years): 9 to 11 hours
- Teenagers (14 to 17 years): 8 to 10 hours
- Adults (18 to 64 years): 7 to 9 hours
- Older adults (over 65 years): 7 to 8 hours

A lack of sleep is a huge factor when it comes to talking about stress on the body. But the flip side to this is that everyday life stressors can interrupt our sleep patterns because of thoughts whirring around in our head, not allowing us to get relaxed enough to fall asleep. It's that chicken or egg again, right?

Many times we tend to rely on quick over-the-counter medications to help us relieve our sleep issues. Instead, your aim should be to maximize your relaxation techniques before heading to bed. Here are some tips:

- Make your bedroom tranquil with no reminders of stressors, no electronics (at least an hour before bedtime)
- Avoid caffeine and excessive alcohol during the evening
- Start to unwind and calm your mind before going to bed
- Try taking a warm, relaxing bath
- Reading a book for fun, not related to work
- Go to bed at the same time and have the same bedtime routine each day

As Jim Rohn says, "Take care of your body. It's the only place you have to live!"

Chapter 8

Step 5 – Opportunities for Internal Growth

"Strength and growth come only through continuous effort and struggle."

– Napoleon Hill

There are so many factors above and beyond the everyday physical lifestyle changes we know we need to change. A lot of times the things that are standing in our way are the internal battles that we have going on. A friend of mine who is a social worker described her own life at one point as feeling like "A pilot light that has been out for so long." If we ignore our feelings and we don't allow ourselves to feel and try to figure out the underlying causes or thoughts, it can adversely affect your health. When we feel this way, our body responds. We have all heard of the "fight or flight" concept. When our bodies and minds are in constant turmoil and struggling with issues, our body elicits a stress response. This will be discussed in greater detail in the next chapter. Right now, we are going to talk about the things that cause this response to happen.

Personal Relationships

We have relationships with our parents, spouse, kids, friends, and even ourselves. Where we struggle most of the time is being able to set boundaries in all of these relationships. Letting people know what you need to have happen to help you and your health. The other piece to all of this is being able to say the dreaded two letter word – *No!* Knowing when to say no to something that is not a necessity or not something vitally important to yours or your family's life. Now, I'll be honest, I myself have an extremely difficult time with both things – setting boundaries and saying no. I always find that when I do practice these, it can come back and bite me if I let it. So, it's about knowing why you are doing what you are doing and feeling good about your decision regardless of the outcome and how the other person ends up reacting.

Another theory to think about is this quote by Jim Rohn: "We are the average of the five people we spend the most time with." As human beings we are heavily influenced, whether we like it or not, by the people we surround ourselves with. It affects our thoughts, our self-esteem, and the decisions we make. Yes, everyone is their own person, but research has shown that we're more affected by our environment than we think. There are two ways to look at this theory (1) surround yourself with positive people that lift you up constantly, or (2) surround yourself with a mixture of positive and negative people that help you make progress in your life – take the negative and rise above it and make yourself stronger.

Professional/Career Life

As a woman, I feel that a majority of us at one point or another have struggled with: What should I be doing – wife, mom, career woman? It goes back to the idea of harmony. Figuring out what we want and how that fits into our current life situations. Figuring out what our passions are and aligning that with our purpose. After doing some research with a group of women ages ranged from twenty-five to forty-five, these are just some of the questions they are asking themselves:

- Did you pick the right career path? If not, is it OK to switch?
- Does your chosen career align with your purpose?
- Do you wake up every morning feeling like you are doing what *sets your soul on fire*?
- Is it OK to take time off to spend time with your family or figure out what it is you really want to do?
- Does it really matter what other people think about your career choices?

For example, my social worker friend, in my opinion, was doing amazing things to help people with their lives already. However, she felt like she should be doing more *good* for this world. The lack of energy and diminishing health and stress were way too much. But after re-evaluating her career and seeing that there are several other ways to make the world a better place in her own special way, she feels more at peace with decisions she has made.

Financial Wellness

I am no accountant, but I have always had a good sense about money and savings and the basic concepts of financial wellness. I know that if you are struggling to make ends meet or have a different concept about this subject than your partner, there will be added struggles and stress on you and your relationship(s).

Financial problems are consistently rated among the highest source of stress for people, and can cause anxiety, frustration and feelings of hopelessness. Financial stress that many endure can lead to health problems, such as trouble sleeping, less focus, moodiness and generally feeling run-down. The combination of stress, anxiety and lack of sleep can lower your immune system and cause more colds and minor illnesses and can also worsen existing medical conditions. More than that, those with financial problems are more likely to neglect their own healthcare and self-care, such as not spending money on preventative care or not taking medication and treatment regimens for chronic conditions properly. Over time, all of the above factors can increase the likelihood of an unhealthy lifestyle and higher medical bills.

Talking more specifically about women, we tend to have so many stresses when it comes to our professional life, but the top question that keeps coming up is: How can I make money doing what I love? Women are looking to feel empowered by the work they do and are looking for ways to make money and enjoy what they do – thereby decreasing the daily stress of having/wanting to work. We all want to feel that we have the ability, knowledge and emotional strength to deal with student-loan debt, rising costs of living, and being able to negotiate a raise. As more people align themselves with the full 360-degree view of wellness, confidence in your finances becomes a huge part of the health and wellness puzzle.

Spirituality

"Happiness is when what you Think, what you Say, and what you Do are in harmony."
– Mahatma Gandhi

The apparent connection between your mind, body, and spirit is seen when one of these areas is affected and we just can't seem to have harmony in our lives. If you are wanting to improve on this area in your life, first thing to keep in mind is that we are all different, so one thing that works for one person, may not work for you. Find what feels right and is comfortable for you.

- Identify things in your life that bring you inner peace, strength, love, comfort, and connection.
- Make time each day to do things that help you spiritually. No matter what your belief is – the connection to a higher purpose as to why you are

here on this planet is so important to how we handle our everyday stresses.

- Examples of what you can do to connect: community service or volunteering, meditation, praying, reading inspirational books, quiet time, yoga, playing a sport you enjoy, or religious services.
- Another practice that we will talk about later in this book is *gratitude*! Having gratitude for everything that we do have is key to not dwelling on the things we don't.

Mindset

One of my favorite books on this subject is called "Mindset: The New Psychology of Success" by Carol S. Dweck. She says, "Fear makes us defensive when we live in a fixed mindset, but it makes us adaptive in the growth mindset." Do you have a fixed mindset or a growth mindset? To find out, let's explain what each of these is:

- *Fixed Mindset* – A person believes that their inherent nature, intelligence, and talents are fixed traits and can't be changed – it's just who they are. This person also believes that her/his talents alone can create success, without any effort.

- *Growth Mindset* – A person believes anyone can be good at something with practice/ effort/ and hard work.
- Below is a table with examples of each type of mindset:

Fixed Mindset	Growth Mindset
Fear of being judged or labeled a failure (tend to hide flaws)	Flaws are just another to-do item of things to improve
Confidence is built from what you already know	Confidence is boosted by continuously improving what you don't know and pushing past the comfort zone (always learning)
Believing that passion and purpose is an inherent thing inside you	Believing that passion and purpose come from discovery, expertise and experience; continuously mastering skills and gaining knowledge
Failures define you	Failures are temporary setbacks
Everything is about the outcome; Failure equals effort wasted	Everything is about the process, the outcome doesn't matter (i.e., "fail forward")

Ultimately, according to Carol Dweck, "No matter what your ability is, effort is what ignites that ability and turns it into accomplishment."

Some other things that can get in the way of our having a growth mindset is also how much input of information and tasks we put in our brain all day long! *We* are a society that loves to be busy, and let's face it continuously pile things onto our plates daily. Let's take me for example: I am a wife, a mom of two young boys, I am extremely involved in both of their schools, I help my aging parents as much as I can (plus I try to spend as much time with them as I can), I run four facets to my business, I have a social life (when I can), and then amidst all of this I have to find time for self-care. Sound familiar? We all have the same twenty-four hours in a day and no matter how hard we try to make it thirty-two hours, it's still only twenty-four. How do we make all of this happen and keep a growth mindset? We find simple tools to use throughout the day, here is a list of some of the things I have to do to keep it all straight:

- Nightly brain dumps
- Setting up a priorities system
  - Traditionally, I am a pen and paper kind of girl. OK, who am I kidding, Office Supply stores are

my version of a toy store! But I have decided to join the 21st century and have found systems and processes to put into place that use a healthy mix of both the old-fashioned way and technology.

- Keeping things organized in my house & structured for all aspects of my and my family's life.
- Detailed scheduling and using the calendar to my advantage
  - Time blocking
  - Preparing the week ahead and prep for the next day the night before
- And last, but certainly not least, keeping a positive attitude at the forefront of my mind.

How Does Positive Thinking Affect Your Life?

We are not ostriches; positive thinking doesn't mean that you bury your head in the sand and ignore life's tough or unpleasant situations. Positive thinking means that you approach hard times in a more positive and productive way.

How we talk to ourselves (self-talk) is where we need to start with positive thinking. Self-talk is automatically running thoughts through our head all day long that can be positive or negative. Some of your self-talk comes from logic but a lot of times it comes from the stories we make up in our head or from the lack of information we have. When it comes to our health, that lack of information can definitely lead to a downward spiral because we can't understand why certain things aren't working for us.

As I have been working on my own life and health recently, I learned about a few stories that I had completely made up from things that were happening around me as a child. No one ever said anything to me about certain situations; it was all my observations and interpretation of what I thought I should be doing. More than that, I carried those stories with me for many years. When I sit back and reflect on that, I see how it has impacted my life both positive and negative in so many ways. The key is awareness. Every time you have a negative thought, stop and ask yourself where it came from and notice how it has affected your life. This is how we stop these patterns. Heading toward addressing those stories and more positive thinking can have some great benefits for your health!

Health Benefits of Positive Thinking

According to researchers at the Mayo Clinic, these are some of the health benefits that positive thinking can provide:

- Increased life span
- Lower rates of depression
- Lower levels of distress
- Greater resistance to the common cold
- Better psychological and physical well-being
- Better cardiovascular health and reduced risk of death from cardiovascular disease
- Better coping skills during hardships and times of stress

A couple of theories as to why having positive thoughts can render health benefits is you tend to cope better with stressful situations, which reduces the harmful health effects of stress on your body, and positive people tend to lead healthier lifestyles (i.e., more physical activity, healthier diet, and don't smoke or drink alcohol in excess).

Tips to Create the New Habit of Positive Thinking

- Identify areas to change
  - Think about an area in your life that you tend to have more negative emotions toward (i.e., work, a relationship). Start by training your brain to think in a more positive way until that situation can change.

- Check yourself regularly
  - o Stop and evaluate what you're thinking about throughout the day. If most of your thoughts are negative, find a way to put a positive spin on them.
- Find humor
  - o Give yourself permission to smile or laugh during difficult times. Laughter helps ease the stress factor.
- Follow a healthy lifestyle
  - o Exercise can positively affect mood and reduce stress. A healthy diet can fuel your mind and body. Managing stress will be discussed further in the next chapter.
- Surround yourself with positive people
  - o Negative people can increase your stress level and make you doubt who you are.
- Practice positive self-talk
  - o One simple rule: Don't say anything to yourself that you wouldn't say to anyone else.

CHAPTER 9:

Step 6 – Nurture Your Stress Relief

"The day she let go of the things that were weighing her
down, was the day she began to shine the brightest."

– Katrina Mayer

When our body is in acute stress mode, it produces a "fight or flight" response. The body's response to this type of stress activates the sympathetic nervous system by a sudden release of hormones from the adrenal glands, adrenaline and noradrenaline. This response can happen with the threat of physical danger or a psychological threat (i.e., having to give a big presentation).

When stress occurs, many hormones are released such as epinephrine and norepinephrine, overproduction of glucose, glucagon, growth hormone, and the number one stress hormone cortisol. Cortisol has beneficial effects at normal levels and is produced to help control certain body functions. Cortisol prepares the body for the fight or flight response by stimulating extra glucose as energy for the large muscles. Cortisol slows insulin production to prevent glucose from being stored so it can be used right away. Cortisol narrows the arteries while the epinephrine increases heart rate, to help blood pump harder and faster. And after the initial threat is gone – the hormone levels drop back down to normal.

The problem occurs, when the cortisol hormone is constantly present in our ever-stressed, fast-paced lifestyles, which wreaks havoc on our health. Let me explain how this can happen:

- Blood Sugar Imbalance/Insulin Resistance/Diabetes
  - Since cortisol increases the amount of glucose in the body to ward off a threat, and in turn suppresses insulin production and release (the main hormone to decrease the amount of blood sugar in the blood stream) – the chronic effect leads to higher blood sugar levels and insulin resistance in the body. Over time, the pancreas struggles to keep up with the high demand for insulin, glucose levels in the blood stay high, the

cells can't get the sugar they need, and the cycle continues. All pointing in the direction of Type 2 Diabetes.

- Weight Gain/Obesity
    - o Cortisol moves triglycerides from storage to visceral fat storage (in the abdomen). Cortisol is also used in the development of mature fat cells.
    - o The consistently high blood glucose levels along with insulin suppression can leave cells starved of glucose and begging for energy. The main way to fix this problem is to send hunger signals to the brain. This can lead to overeating and unused glucose which leads to it being stored as fat.
    - o Cortisol also plays a role in appetite and cravings of high caloric foods by binding to the hypothalamus receptors in the brain.
- Immune System Suppression
    - o Cortisol can reduce inflammation but with chronic cortisol, over time the attempt to reduce inflammation can wreak havoc on the immune system which can lead to a whole host of problems (i.e., increased susceptibility to colds and other viruses, autoimmune disease)

- Gastrointestinal Problems
  - As we stated before, when cortisol is being produced, the sympathetic nervous system is being activated, thereby suppressing the parasympathetic nervous system (PNS). The PNS is what aids in eating and digestion in the body. So, while this is being suppressed, digestion and absorption are compromised, indigestion develops, and the mucosal lining of the GI tract becomes irritated and inflamed. And this inflammation causes increased production of cortisol – the vicious cycle continues.
- Cardiovascular Problems
  - In acute stress, cortisol constricts blood vessels and increases blood pressure to allow for enhanced oxygenated blood flow. However, over time artery constriction and high blood pressure leads to vessel damage and plaque buildup – the prime environment for a heart attack.
- Fertility Problems:
  - Continuous elevation of cortisol can lead to erectile dysfunction and disruption in ovulation and menstruation. Also, androgenic sex hormones are produced in the adrenal glands

where cortisol and epinephrine are produced. So, over production of cortisol can decrease the production of these sex hormones.

What is inflammation?

Stress can cause inflammation in the body, so we are going to first talk about what inflammation really is. There are two main types of inflammation Acute vs. Chronic.

- Acute inflammation (also known as "healthy inflammation") is a short-term defense mechanism. It is how your body responds to immediate damage to tissues and helps start the healing process. (i.e., when you get a cut or scrape, acute inflammation occurs when the white blood cells rush to the site and prevent damage from spreading to other tissues and fights off foreign invaders.)
- Chronic inflammation (also known as "unhealthy inflammation") is long-term stress on the body and can cause widespread damage throughout the body and trigger a whole host of devastating conditions.

We will be focusing on discussing the effects of chronic inflammation and how this comes about in our bodies.

Chronic inflammation occurs when the cells in our bodies are stressed by different factors both internal and external. It can also happen when the body thinks there is a foreign invader that really is not there. When an inflammatory response like this is triggered and there is not a true foreign substance, the reaction stays there, it lingers around and wreaks havoc on the surrounding tissues and cells. Unfortunately, this type of response can linger around for a long time, going unnoticed. This is called "low-grade" chronic inflammation. Left untreated over time, chronic inflammation can create many significant threats to our bodies and minds (i.e., autoimmune diseases, cognitive decline (dementia), heart disease, and Type 2 Diabetes, etc.)

Are you Chronically Inflamed? – Quiz:

1. Do you feel fatigued even when you have had sufficient sleep?
2. Do you experience bouts of "brain fog," depression, anxiety on a regular basis?
3. Do you experience a lowered sex drive?
4. Do you feel like you are constantly getting sick and susceptible to seasonal illnesses (i.e. your immune system isn't working like it should)?
5. Do you get frequent allergy symptoms?

6. Have you been diagnosed with an autoimmune disorder (i.e., Hashimoto's, IBD, Arthritis, Lupus, etc.)?

7. Have you been told you have metabolic syndrome (i.e. your typical blood work results are off – blood sugar, cholesterol, blood pressure, body measurements)?

8. Do your joints feel puffy or swollen, or do you feel bloated all over throughout the day?

9. Do you have digestive issues on a regular basis?

10. Do you have frequent skin breakouts or issues?

If you said yes to any of these questions, and especially if you said yes to many of these questions, then you are quite possibly experiencing chronic inflammation and your body has been trying to tell you this for a while.

We have talked about the negative effects on the body due to chronic stress and the continuous release of stress hormones like cortisol and the inflammation that ensues – let's now talk about what that has translated to in our society.

Research that was presented at the American College of Cardiology's 68th Scientific Session in March 2019, suggests that it's time for younger people to take notice of their heart health. Dr. Ron Blankstein, the study's senior author, reports, "1 in every 5 people who suffers from a heart attack is 40 years old or younger, and overall the average rate of heart attacks in that age group has increased at a rate of 2 percent per year between 2006 and 2016." Heart attacks can be prevented, so why is it that the age group for this occurrence is getting younger and younger? The answer is *stress*, which leads to inflammation! In my opinion, it's because we spend so much time as a society running around and piling things on our to-do lists that we don't stop and take time for self-care, stress reduction, and we complain of less time, and want way more convenience. Anxiety and depression are also on the rise today. The initial thought in a society of convenience is there is a pill for those conditions. It feels like every other commercial shows us that. In my opinion, we don't *necessarily* need medications to stop the anxiety and depression that can ensue from stress in our everyday lives. There are many ways to help us cope with the everyday stressors and the feelings of anxiety and depression. I feel that a lot of people rely on antidepressants solely because they've been prescribed, and they don't work on figuring out and fixing the actual issue. I also believe there are some circumstances that may warrant short-term use (i.e. death of a family member) or long-term use (i.e. diagnosed mental illness) of these types of prescriptions. I know several people who have been able to use these medications as a bridge to get to the other side of the situation and come off them. But before making any changes to any medication regimen please *always* consult with your physician or pharmacist.

So, what are the lifestyle factors that can trigger or worsen chronic inflammation? Obesity, insufficient sleep, smoking, excessive alcohol intake, illicit drug use, poor nutrition, excessive or incorrect exercise habits, and consistently elevated stress levels. Many of these factors have been discussed in previous chapters, but the one that often gets overlooked is the idea of *stress*, also known as "the silent killer." Stress is a known contributor to high blood pressure, cardiovascular disease and stomach disorders, among other conditions.

Techniques/ Tips for Stress Management:

- Avoid caffeine, alcohol, and nicotine (caffeine and nicotine are stimulants and can increase stress levels; alcohol in large amounts acts as a depressant, and in smaller quantities acts as a stimulant – increasing stress levels)
- Physical activity (i.e. yoga, twenty-minute walk, dance session) can metabolize the excess stress hormones
- Rest

- Healthy nutrition
- Relaxation techniques (i.e. meditation, guided imagery)
- Talking to someone (i.e. a counselor, or get social support)
- Journaling
- Time management
- Learn to say no

In addition to taking inventory of your lifestyle, there are several blood tests that can be done to check for markers of inflammation and other disorders that may be going on. There are also several herbs and supplements that can be recommended to help you on your journey to decreasing the inflammation. Talk to a holistic healthcare practitioner to help guide you in the right direction with the right information for you.

CHAPTER 10:

Step 7 – You Have the P.O.W.E.R!

"We are what we repeatedly do.
Excellence, then, is not an act, but a habit."
– Aristotle

Any time we talk about a health and wellness journey, in order to get the lasting transformative results we are looking for, the bottom line is we have to make *lasting* lifestyle changes. I am here to share that *You* have the P-O-W-E-R to do this for yourself in order to live the healthy life of your dreams. Here is a process I came up with and have used with several patients of mine, including myself, with great results and who were able to maintain the healthy lifestyles they wanted. You will want to get a notebook and on the side of the first page write the acronym P.O.W.E.R. Next to each letter, write the description in your own life of what the prompt is telling you to do, then each day also go into this journal and write out your feelings of how things went for this problem on a daily basis:

P – Problem: Choose a habit/problem to change.

O – Overall Goal: Write down what the overall goal is and why this change would be good.

W – What: Think of a way(s) to make the change happen. What are you going to do? How long will you do it? (I recommend a week at a time.)

E – Evaluate: Could you do it each day for the time period you specified?

R – Reward: Celebrate success! (I do not recommend using food as a reward – that just begs to send you into a downward spiral. Suggestions – a new outfit, a movie, a fun excursion with friends, a massage)

Practice this change and new habit for a week and evaluate where you are. Do you need to continue working on this one thing or has it become easy to manage? You will work on this one habit until it becomes second nature for you and then continue to the next habit to change (while maintaining the habits you have already been working on). Before you know it, you will have changed several habits and start to realize how amazing you are starting to feel.

Along with the daily P-O-W-E-R habit changes, journaling can be such a huge benefit to you on your health journey.

The Power of Journaling

One of my favorite books is called *The Miracle Morning*, by Hal Elrod. He says, "Writing in a journal each day, with a structured, strategic process allows you to direct your focus to what you did accomplish, what you're grateful for, and what you're committed to doing better tomorrow. Thus, you more deeply enjoy your journey each day, feel good about any forward progress you made, and use a heightened level of clarity to accelerate your results."

Benefits of Journaling:

- Reduce stress
- Gather and explain your thoughts and feelings
- Discover more about yourself- uncover what makes you happy, what drives you, and how to effectively navigate your emotions and behaviors
- Work through difficult feelings and learning to self-soothe

- Solve problems through critical thinking and using our emotions, intuition, and creativity
- Practice forgiveness and reflect on disagreements, and cultivate understanding and compassion for others
- Stay accountable to your goals and track improvement (of both short-term and long-term goals)

Tips for Best Journaling Practices:
- Be Yourself – a journal is where you can be your true self without worry of what others may think, be true to yourself and authentic; open up
- Don't worry about spelling and grammar (success = being legible and you can understand it)
- Write by hand (improves your memory recall of events and what you have written)

Three Important Things to Include:
- Gratitude:
  - This is the simplest, most effective thing you can do every day to be happier.
  - Gratitude is the practice of counting one's blessings.

o Let's get into the science of why gratitude is the closest thing to a "magic pill" for happiness. In a 2008 study, *The Neural Basis of Human Social Values*, subjects experiencing gratitude were studied using functional Magnetic Resonance Imaging (fMRI). It was found that they were influencing their hypothalamus in real time. The hypothalamus is a part of your brain that plays a role in sleep, eating and stress. Gratitude also stimulates the neurotransmitter dopamine (known as the "feel-good" hormone).

o To-Do: List out three things you are grateful for to start off your day

o Bonus: List out three things you are grateful for at the end of your day (right before bed)

• Free Writing:

o Be free and write whatever comes to mind, don't establish any rules.

o Being able to openly express what is going on in your life at the present moment and how you are feeling without judgement is the greatest benefit to journaling.

o To-Do: Do this practice in the evening and follow with Positive Thinking exercise below.

- Positive Thinking:
  - This is the best way to cultivate optimism in your day!
  - Every thought releases some type of chemical. When you have positive thoughts and you are feeling happy/ optimistic, cortisol (stress hormone) decreases and the brain produces serotonin, creating a feeling of well-being. In a paper written in 2017 by A. Scaccia, she explains that, when serotonin levels are normal, one feels happy, calmer, less anxious, more focused, and more emotionally stable. Dopamine is also released which helps control the brain's reward system and pleasure center.
  - To-Do: List three amazing things that happened to you during the day. It can be as big as getting a promotion at work to the small things like getting a hug from a loved one.

Your P-O-W-E-R lies within you. This quote by Jillian Michaels sums it all up, "It's not about perfect. It's about effort. And when you bring that every single day, that's where the transformation happens. That's how change occurs."

CHAPTER 11:

Now Is the Time to Lead the Life of Your Dreams

"Health is not valued until sickness comes."

– Thomas Fuller

Sometimes we feel just fine and our bloodwork is off. Sometimes we feel awful and our bloodwork is just fine. Or maybe we feel awful and our bloodwork is off as well. No matter which path you fit into – don't wait until you are sick to value your health.

The process is laid out for you, now what? Information is all around us and the phrase "knowledge is power" is out there for a reason. But not all information is created equal. We have talked a lot about that in this book. So, where do you begin? What resources are reputable? What information applies to you?

Yes, you have tried what you feel like is everything under the sun to bring down those blood work results and to feel better. The one thing that you haven't tried is figuring out what is right for *You*. Now is *not* the time to give up, *now is the time* to shift gears and focus on you! Knowledge is power if you have the information about you and your history, your life and your own body.

Let's imagine building a house: would you start by (A) building a solid (cemented) foundation and then start putting up the wooden beams to create walls, or (B) start with the wooden beams and maybe decide later to go back and lay the cement under it if necessary? Personally, I would choose *A* and start with a solid foundation and the knowledge that everything I do that comes after will work and not come crashing down.

What usually ends up happening when you start on a health journey – you do well for a while and if you aren't seeing the results you want, or something shinier comes along we stop and move in another direction.

Not having control of your health can be such a huge detriment to not only you but the loved ones around you. You know my health journey story – but let me tell you how I had been feeling throughout that whole process. I felt unhealthy, out of control, like a failure in all the aspects of my life from being an effective wife, mom, daughter, professional, and friend. I was constantly scared of losing my life early because I wasn't able to have control over my numbers and how my health was going. I felt like I was killing myself to do the right thing and never felt like I knew what the right thing was. I can tell you from my experience that living a life in fear is no way to live your life. Every day I felt like I was building the walls to my health, but with absolutely no foundation. You have to do things in the right order to be effective and get the strong, lasting results you want.

My kids are eight and five years old and I have spent a majority of this time thinking about what I should do next for my health. I spent more time worrying about the issue and searching for the wrong answers instead of actually taking care of myself. Even when I was doing activities of self-care, my mind was always somewhere else, like I should be spending time with my kids or some other feeling of guilt. The problem with that is when I was with my kids, my mind would be on something else I should be doing like work or self-care to take care of my health. It was a lose-lose situation in my opinion. It took me a long time and a lot of lost years to figure out that what I really needed to do was do things in the right way. All the things I did were not a waste, but they were not as effective as they could have been. What I learned was that without doing things in the right order and with the right, individualized information for me and building my health from the ground up, there was no way to get over the fear of a less effective or shorter life. Putting myself through the 7 Steps to H.A.R.M.O.N.Y. has brought my life back. I know that having a guide to be a part of your support system to hold you accountable and help you see the forest through the trees can be the most beneficial thing you do. It may just save your life!

CHAPTER 12:

You Are Not Alone

"Looking after your health today, gives you hope for a better tomorrow. Walking this journey with someone beside you gives your life the harmony that it needs."

– Asha Pai Bohannon

I have gone through so much to find answers. I have spent so many years telling my family "I wish I could find a *me* for *me!* Someone willing to take the time to look at me as a whole person and ask the questions that need to be asked and see me through the *entire* process!" I finally decided to be my own *me* for *me!*

So, just like that, I want you to feel empowered and not to give up on yourself. I want you to not swim in an ocean with massive waves that you don't know how to navigate and then end up wiping out time and time again. My desire is for you to find the right person to help you on your journey that will take the time you need to look at you as an individual and hold your hand through this process so that by the end you can "spread your wings" in transformation and lead the healthy life of your dreams with your blood work back to normal and the feeling that you can do anything you want to do. Let me give you an example that comes to my mind about getting the right kind of help – your yearly taxes. You can absolutely get a computer program and figure out how to file your taxes on your own. You may or may not get it right; you may or may not put in all the things you need to. A lot of the times you save it until the last minute, because, let's face it, it may not be a top priority and you have a million other things to focus on. However, if you hire a tax professional, you are confident that the job will get done in the manner it should be. Things will not get missed; in fact he/she may find things that you would have missed. Hiring this tax professional, whose main focus is preparing taxes, you are guaranteed a more in-depth performance. Aren't you worth that?

It's the same thing with your health: remember that you *are* worth the time and energy for someone to help you with your health issues. We have become a society of quick fixes – and while prescription medications may be necessary at times – with the right resources and knowledge, they may not always be the answer. Our bodies are meant to heal on their own if we give it the proper care and things it needs from food and nutrition (including supplements), and self-care we can find the right ways to heal ourselves. Looking at the whole person as an individual is what the healthcare system is missing.

Yes, as a pharmacist, I know there is a place for prescription medications, but it doesn't have to be the first go-to. Often times more problems arise from it, and the more and more that is added, the worse they can make you feel. The missing link is people taking the time with you. Complaints are taken as "you are the problem" and moves to what quick fix can be given to "appease" you ("band-aid" society).

I learned a concept during my years in pharmacy school called pharmaceutical care. It means to treat patients with compassion, be willing to listen, and be willing to dig deeper. Many practitioners display an "out of sight, out of mind" manner and don't give the follow-up and accountability piece that is necessary when working through lifestyle and habit changes.

For many years in my practice, I have often seen that the right hand doesn't necessarily know what the left hand is doing. We doctor/practitioner hop, we pharmacy hop, and many people don't even know what it all means or how to put it all together. It has been quite the challenge to find that one place you can go to have someone educate you on what is right for you, and inspire you to do better, and help you advocate for yourself. My wish for you is to find the support and compassion you need to become your own patient healthcare advocate and lead a life full of Health, Hope, and Harmony!

ACKNOWLEDGMENTS

There are several people in my life I want to thank for helping me put this book out into the world. First, my parents. Thank you, Mom and Dad, for continuously supporting me and showing me that I can chase after my dreams by putting one foot in front of the other. Thank you for helping with my kids when I just needed time to write (and all those other times too). Thank you to my husband, Eric, for helping me see what is possible and for believing in me every step of the way. Thank you for holding down the fort when I needed it most! Thank you to my boys, Naveen and Shaleen for bringing the "New Light" into my life and making me want to be your inspiration in this world. Anything is possible with effort and a good, kind heart! I love you all to the moon and back, infinity and beyond and forever and always!

Thank you to the many, many patients that have crossed my path – you all became part of my family as I stepped with you on your health journey and continue to see you soar for many years after. Thank you for opening your world to me and allowing me to help you find *your* answers! It is an honor to get to do what I do daily!

Thank you to Angela Lauria and The Author Incubator's team, as well as to David Hancock and the Morgan James Publishing team for helping me bring this book to print.

THANK YOU

Thank you so much for reading *To Medicate or Not? That Is the Question! The Ultimate Guide to Improving Blood Test Results*. I am incredibly humbled and excited that you made it this far! Making it to this point in the book means that you are ready to move your health in a new direction and know that it isn't a one-size-fits-all journey.

Firstly, I would love to learn more about your journey up to this point. I would love for you to keep in touch and share your stories, find me at:

Website: ashapaibohannon.com
Email: asha@ashapaibohannon.com
Facebook: www.facebook.com/drashapaibohannon
Instagram: instagram.com/dr.ashapaibohannon

Secondly, I am so passionate about patient advocacy and you getting the information that is right for you and your body. Send an email to asha@ashapaibohannon.com for a free video class on how to start 7 Steps to H.A.R.M.O.N.Y.™ and getting on the right track to living a healthier, happier life that you have always dreamed of.

Thank you again for supporting me and my passion for helping you find the resources and information that are right for you and allowing me to inspire you along your health journey!

About the Author

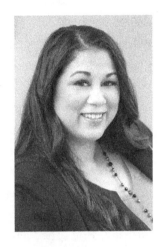

Dr. Asha Pai Bohannon is a holistic health guide. As a Doctor of Pharmacy with multiple health certifications, including diabetes education, medication therapy management, personal training, and more, she is passionate about sharing her best resources for helping you lead a healthier, happier life. She graduated from University of North Carolina at Chapel Hill in 2002 and has spent over fifteen years helping over 1,200 patients find their own ways to take control of their own health and wellness.

After having suffered with being a "medical mystery" for so many years, she decided to take matters into her own hands and start treating herself like she has the thousands of other patients that have come across her path.

To learn more about her complete wellness solutions, explore her signature program, 7 Steps to H.A.R.M.O.N.Y.™, through her wellness practice. Patient Advocacy Initiative (PAI) Wellness Group is a holistic health practice for individuals and corporate organizations. For those seeking growth opportunities and healthy skincare, allow her to help you as a recognized leader with Rodan + Fields, a dermatology-based skincare company. She loves walking alongside her patients to help them identify and define the roles medications and other resources should play in leading them to healthy lives they can fully enjoy. Let her help you find your best path as you work together to create your fresh start!

Some other passions she has is in her partnership with her husband, Eric. They have a thriving business helping other people (specifically health care practitioners) get started with new entrepreneurial businesses through business strategy and mentoring. She also loves coaching other Moms on tactical strategies to find what *sets their soul on fire* and begin to live their lives with passion and purpose- while *slaying life* and all that comes with being the WOMAN they want to be!

Dr. Asha lives in Raleigh, North Carolina with her husband and two sons. Her private practice is available for private consultations in person or via phone or video conferencing.

9 781642 798241